漫画中药故事系列
# Chinese Medicines in Cartoon Series

# 品读中药
（汉英对照）
## Tales of Food and TCM
(Chinese-English)

杨柏灿　主编
**Edited by** Yang Baican

杨熠文　晋　永　鲍思思　祝建龙　◎**文/译**
**Paperwork by** Yang Yiwen, Jin Yong, Bao Sisi, Zhu Jianlong

孔珏莹　夏瑜桢　金潇逸　◎**绘**
**Brushwork by** Kong Jueying, Xia Yuzhen, Jin Xiaoyi

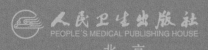
人民卫生出版社
PEOPLE'S MEDICAL PUBLISHING HOUSE
·北　京·

**图书在版编目（CIP）数据**

品读中药：汉英对照 / 杨柏灿主编 . —北京：人民卫生出版社，2021.3

（漫画中药故事系列）

ISBN 978-7-117-31335-3

I. ①品… II. ①杨… III. ①中药材 – 普及读物 – 汉、英 IV. ①R282-49

中国版本图书馆 CIP 数据核字（2021）第 038064 号

| 人卫智网 | www.ipmph.com | 医学教育、学术、考试、健康，购书智慧智能综合服务平台 |
| --- | --- | --- |
| 人卫官网 | www.pmph.com | 人卫官方资讯发布平台 |

**漫画中药故事系列——品读中药（汉英对照）**

Manhua Zhongyao Gushi Xilie——Pindu Zhongyao（Han-Ying Duizhao）

主　　编：杨柏灿

出版发行：人民卫生出版社（中继线 010-59780011）

地　　址：北京市朝阳区潘家园南里 19 号

邮　　编：100021

E - mail：pmph @ pmph.com

购书热线：010-59787592　010-59787584　010-65264830

印　　刷：北京顶佳世纪印刷有限公司

经　　销：新华书店

开　　本：889×1194　1/24　印张：2.5

字　　数：73 千字

版　　次：2021 年 3 月第 1 版

印　　次：2021 年 4 月第 1 次印刷

标准书号：ISBN 978-7-117-31335-3

定　　价：46.00 元

# 序言

# Foreword

由上海中医药大学杨柏灿教授主编的《漫画中药故事系列》由人民卫生出版社出版了。这也是杨教授十年来从事中医药文化研究、作品创作和开展中医药文化普及工作的又一力作。

中医药是中国优秀传统文化的代表，凝聚着深邃的中国古代哲学智慧和科学文明的精髓。在抗击新冠肺炎疫情中，中医药发挥了突出的作用，引起世人的高度关注。国家的重视、社会的认同和关注，使中医药的发展迎来了前所未有的大好时机。抓住这一千载难逢的契机，做好中医药的传承与创新、推广与普及工作，是每一位中医药工作者义不容辞的责任。

做好中医药的传承、创新与弘扬，首先重在传承，只有真正做好传承，将中医药的精气神传承下来，才有可能不断创新、发展、弘扬。要做好中医药的传承，除了专业院校的教学以及师承以外，在全社会开展中医药知识的普及推广是一项十分重要的工作，特别是重视"从娃娃抓起"，从小就让我们的孩子沐浴中医药知识的阳光雨露，领略中医药世界的奥秘，感受中国传统文化的伟大，树立文化自信，使之入心入脑，有助于增强孩子们的民族自豪感，激发爱国情怀。

*Chinese Medicines in Cartoon Series* compiled by Professor Yang Baican from Shanghai University of Traditional Chinese Medicine (SHTCM) is published by People's Medical Publishing House. It is a masterpiece by Professor Yang after his 10-year study on, writing about and popularization of Chinese medicine culture.

Traditional Chinese medicine (TCM) is representative of traditional Chinese culture, where lies the wisdom of ancient Chinese philosophy and the essence of scientific civilization. In the fight against COVID-19 epidemic, TCM has been playing an important role and attracts a lot of attention. Valued by the nation and accepted and followed with interest by the society, TCM has an unprecedented opportunity for development. It is a duty for every TCM worker to seize this opportunity and perform well in inheritance, innovation, promotion and popularization of TCM.

To inherit, innovate and carry forward TCM, inheritance is the first and foremost. TCM can be innovated, developed and carried forward only when it is inherited properly with its essence handed down. For inheritance of TCM, besides teachings in professional schools and from a master to his/her apprentices, it is important to popularize TCM knowledge in the whole society, with focus on "Starts with children". Let our children bathe in the sunshine of TCM knowledge, get to know the mystery of TCM and feel the magnificence of traditional Chinese culture, so that they can have cultural confidence, which helps enhance their sense of national pride and inspire their love for the country.

近年来，一些有识之士已开展了卓有成效的"中医药走进中小学"的工作，受到了广泛的关注和认同。伴随着国家综合实力的增强，我国国际社会地位的提升，中医药的国际影响力也日益扩大。重视中医药走向国际，弘扬中国传统文化，不但有利于提升我国文化软实力，而且也有益于中医药为全人类造福。

杨柏灿教授是上海中医药大学从事中药学教学的教师。他在完成中医药的医、教、研工作之余，十年来致力于中医药知识的推广与普及工作，在国内最早开设了中药慕课课程《走近中药》《杏林探宝——带你走进中药》《杏林探宝——认知中药》《中药学》《中药知多少》以及微视频《中药知识——走进中小学》。其中《杏林探宝——认知中药》上线美国 Coursera 平台，受众人群遍及 80 余个国家和地区，学习人数达 10 余万人次。同时，杨教授笔耕不辍，六年来先后出版了中医药通识读本《药缘文化——中药与文化的交融》《药名文化——中药与文化的交融》，连续三年出版了《本草光阴——中药养生文化日历》，在社会上产生一定的影响。

In recent years, men of sight have carried out projects of "Introducing TCM into middle and primary schools", which is widely concerned and approved. With enhancement of the overall national strength and the elevated status of China in the international community, TCM has an increasingly large international influence. Paying attention to international communication of TCM and carrying forward traditional Chinese culture can not only strengthen the cultural soft power of China, but also bring benefit for all mankind.

The author is a professor in Chinese medicines in SHTCM. After finishing his work as a doctor, teacher and researcher in TCM, he has been dedicated to promotion and popularization of TCM knowledge for nearly a decade. He is the first to provide MOOCs on Chinese medicines in China, including *Get Closer to Chinese Medicines*, *Hunt for Treasure in Apricot Grove — Bring You Closer to Chinese Medicines*, *Hunt for Treasure in Apricot Grove — Get to Know Chinese Medicines*, *Traditional Chinese Pharmacology* and *What Do You Know About Chinese Medicines*, as well as a micro video of *Knowledge about Chinese Medicines — Introduced into Middle and Primary Schools*. Among them, *Hunt for Treasure in Apricot Grove — Get to Know Chinese Medicines* is available online on Coursera, with audience from more than 80 countries and regions and learned by over 100,000 person-time. At the same time, Professor Yang has been writing continuously. In recent six years, he has published books on TCM including *Medicine Culture—Blending of Chinese Medicines and Culture* and *Medicine Name Culture—Blending of Chinese Medicines and Culture* and has published *Time and Chinese Materia Medica—Health Culture Calendar with Chinese Medicines*, which has a certain social impact.

《漫画中药故事系列》突破了目前市面上单纯以文字讲中药故事，或是将中药故事与中药知识相割离的作品形式，遍查古籍，选取有史实依据、民众知晓度高、具有深厚中国传统文化底蕴的中药故事，通过生动形象的漫画和精练朴实的语言，讲解中药故事，向世人展示中药知识与中国多元优秀传统文化的交融。读者在赏读本丛书时，不但能了解常用的中药知识，还能在不知不觉中接受中国传统文化的熏陶。本丛书的文字部分采用中英文对照的形式，益于中医药在国际上传播，同时也使中小学生在阅读漫画、接受中医药知识之余，提升英语的阅读能力。

本丛书的出版发行对于中医药的推广、普及势必有一定的促进作用，期待杨柏灿教授团队能不断有新的作品问世。

上海市卫生健康委员会副主任
上海市中医药管理局副局长
上海中医药学会会长
原上海中医药大学副校长

胡鸿毅

2020 年 9 月

*Chinese Medicines in Cartoon Series* gets rid of the layout of telling stories about Chinese medicines in words alone or separating the stories from the knowledge. The author has consulted ancient books and selected the stories that are based on historical facts, well known among people and deeply rooted in traditional Chinese culture. The stories about Chinese medicines are told through vivid cartoons and in simple language. They show the world the blending of knowledge about Chinese medicines with traditional Chinese culture, so that the reader can not only know about Chinese medicines, but also feel the charm of traditional Chinese culture. The text part of the series of books is in both Chinese and English to promote international spread of TCM, and additionally, the students in middle and primary schools can have their English reading ability improved while reading the cartoons and learning about Chinese medicines.

Publishing and distribution of this series of books will surely give an impetus to the promotion and popularization of TCM and I look forward to more works by the team led by Professor Yang Baican.

Deputy director, Shanghai Municipal Health Commission

Deputy director, Shanghai Municipal Administrator of Traditional Chinese Medicine

President, Shanghai Association of Traditional Chinese Medicine

Former vice-president, Shanghai University of Traditional Chinese Medicine

**Hu Hongyi**

Sep, 2020

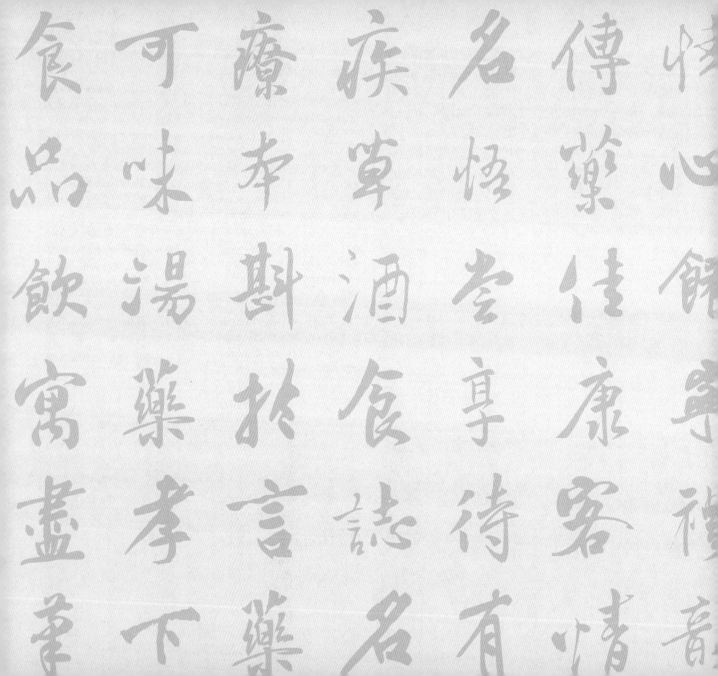

# 前言

# Preface

随着我国综合实力的不断提高和国际地位的日益提升，文化软实力建设、树立文化自信，已成为国家的发展战略。习近平总书记指出"中医药学凝聚着深邃的哲学智慧和中华民族几千年的健康养生理念及其实践经验，是中国古代科学的瑰宝，也是打开中华文明宝库的钥匙"，高屋建瓴地概括了中医药在传统文化中具有不可替代的地位及其所具有的鲜明的文化特征。

《漫画中药故事系列》以历史悠久、扎根于中华大地、深植于大众心灵的中药为切入点，通过具有史料记载、民间知晓度高的典故传说，采用形象生动的漫画形式，传播中药知识，弘扬传统文化。丛书共分四册，既可独立成书又前后互为关联。

第一册《名医药传》：从中药雅称、药物应用、功效发现，介绍家喻户晓的名医名家治疗顽苛痼疾、疑难杂症的故事。

第二册《君药传奇》：从药名来历、药物应用等方面，介绍中药与古代君王间的趣闻典故以及民间医药高手不畏权贵、巧用中药的故事。

With its increasing comprehensive strength and growing status in the world, China's cultural soft power along with cultural confidence turns to renascent tendency. Chinese President Xi Jinping, once claimed that "Traditional Chinese medical theory is the gem of ancient Chinese science and philosophy, and also a key to the treasure of Chinese civilization", reconfirming the irreplaceable position and distinct feature of traditional Chinese medicine (TCM) in our culture.

*Chinese Medicines in Cartoon Series* aims at spreading knowledge of TCM and promoting our national culture. The series takes the well-known herbs as entry, tells fact-based tales and illustrates stories with pictures in comic format. The series includes four books, each being a sub-topic of TCM.

Book I *Tales of Doctors and TCM*: stories about miscellaneous and critical cases, mainly from the aspects of herbs' poetic names and efficacy.

Book II *Tales of Emperors and TCM*: stories about emperors and herbs, mainly from the aspects of herbs' naming and efficacy.

第三册《品读中药》：从汤羹、酒与豆腐发明的故事，介绍中药与饮食文化的渊源，体现药食同源的特性；通过益母草、王不留行、远志等中药名称来历的典故，体现中药药名的文化内涵。

第四册《智用中药》：从药物生长环境、采摘时节、药用部位、应用方式等对药效的影响，体现古今医药学家认识自然、应用自然的智慧。

随着国家对中医药工作日益重视以及在这次抗击新冠肺炎疫情中，中医药不可或缺的作用，重视做好中医药的传承、创新及推广已成为全社会的共识。特别是近年来，越来越多人意识到，要做好中医药的传承应该从小抓起，要重视中医药走进中小学的工作。正是在这样的大背景下，本团队经过 3 年多的努力，在人民卫生出版社的大力支持下，完成了以传播中药知识、弘扬传统文化为宗旨的漫画中药故事系列丛书。期望本丛书的出版发行，能有益于中医药知识和传统文化的传播。

Book III *Tales of Food and TCM*: stories about herbs and diet through the invention of soup, wine and tofu; stories about herbs and its name origin through the naming of motherwort, polygala, etc.

Book IV *Tales of Creative Use and TCM*: stories about herbs and efficacy, mainly from the aspects of herbs' living environment, growing seasons, plant parts and application.

With the increasing emphasis on the traditional Chinese medical theory and its indispensable role in the combat against COVID-19, the whole society has reached the consensus that the traditional Chinese medical theory should be inherited, innovated as well as promoted. In recent years, more and more people have realized that the inheritance of TCM should be cultivated since childhood and that TCM should be introduced into elementary education stage. Thanks to People's Medical Publishing House, our team, after more than three years' constant efforts, has completed this series of comic books on TCM. We are hoping that Chinese medicine and traditional Chinese culture can be promoted after its publication.

考虑到中西方文化背景的不同，在英语翻译上侧重于意译，而非直译，部分内容及标题中英文有所不同，须结合具体故事情节予以理解。

本丛书适用于广大中医药爱好者，特别是中小学生。同时，本丛书中英对照的形式也有助于在国际上传播、宣传中医药知识和中国传统文化，推动中医药国际化。

《漫画中药故事系列》丛书编委会

2020 年 7 月 25 日

Owning to the cultural differences between the East and the West, some parts of the stories have been translated sense-for-sense instead word-for-word.

This series of books is written for Chinese medicine enthusiasts, especially primary and middle school students. Meanwhile, in the form of both Chinese and English, it helps to spread Chinese medicine knowledge and culture so as to promote its internationalization.

Editorial Committee

July 25, 2020

# 目录
## CATALOG

### 第一部分
### 食药之美 |1

煲汤煎药本同源 | 2
百药之长亦佳酿 | 8
无意之举创豆腐 | 14

### Part I
### Enjoying the Good Taste of Medicine | 1

Making Soup and Decocting Medicine | 2
The Invention of Wine | 8
Gypsum and Tofu | 14

# 第二部分
## 寓药之情 |21

母慈子孝益母草 |22

待客之道槟榔礼 |28

闭门逐客王不留 |34

志存高远誉远志 |40

# Part Ⅱ
## The Feelings in the Medicine |21

Motherwort and Filial Piety |22

*Areca catechu* and Courtesy |28

*Vaccaria segetalis* and Deportation Order |34

Polygala and Aspiration |40

# 第一部分
# 食药之美

药与食同源不可分。平日里在煲汤、饮酒、吃菜之时，其实也在品味着我们的中药。

# Part I
# Enjoying the Good Taste of Medicine

Medicine and our daily food share the same origin. In fact, we have been enjoying tasting our traditional Chinese medicine in our soup, wine and dishes.

# 煲汤煎药本同源
## Making Soup and Decocting Medicine

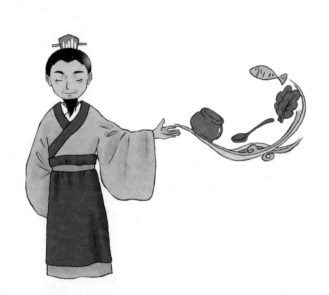

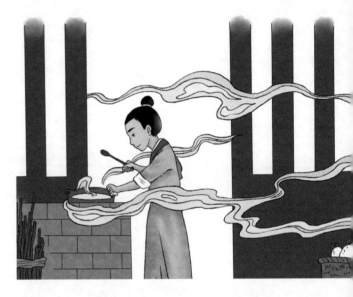

伊尹曾辅佐汤建立商朝，被后人尊奉为中国历史上第一位"贤相"，不过他治国的灵感却是来源于烹调之中。

Yi Yin, who assisted Tang in establishing the Shang Dynasty, was honored with "the first wise prime minister" in Chinese history by later generations. However, his inspiration for governing the country came from cooking.

伊尹年轻时地位卑微，只是一个陪嫁奴隶，在汤的厨房专职烹调。

Yi Yin used to be a humble dowry slave working in the kitchen for the imperial court.

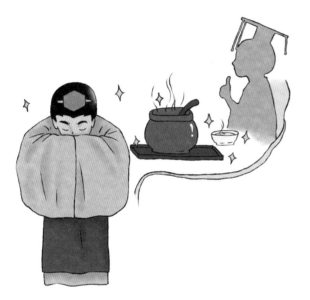

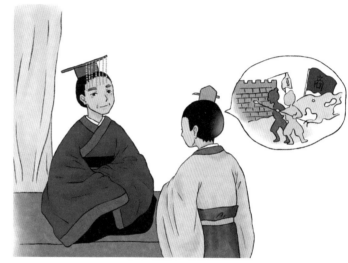

不过，伊尹却精于调和，擅长将各种食材共同煲制成美味的汤羹，而这也因此赢得汤的赏识，被封为御厨。

However, unlike many other common cooks, Yi Yin was good at blending delicious soup by mixing various ingredients, so he won the favor of Tang and earned himself the title of chef.

不仅在烹饪上造诣不凡，伊尹在治国之术上也十分有见地。常借上菜的机会与汤王会面，劝其讨伐夏桀，拯救人民。

Yi Yin had talent not only for cooking, but also for administering the country. Taking his opportunity of food serving for the Emperor Tang, he many a time suggested the emperor save the people by crusading against Emperor Jie of the Xia Dynasty.

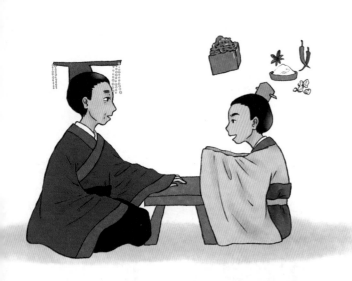

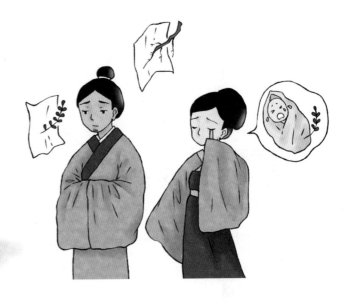

伊尹的才华也逐渐得到了汤的认可。此后，汤常向伊尹询问天下事，伊尹擅长烹饪，便常以做菜比喻引申治国之道。

而在当时，医生的处方多是单味草药，对一些复杂的病情往往药力不够，也常产生毒性反应，药效总是不佳。

Yi Yin's talent had gradually been recognized by Tang. Since then, Tang often asked Yi Yin for advice. As he was good at cooking, Yi Yin often used cooking metaphors to explain the management of state affairs.

At that time, most of the doctors' prescriptions contained only one single herb, which were often ineffective and even toxic to some complicated diseases, so the efficacy was always poor.

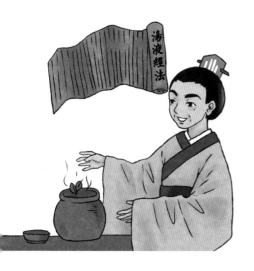
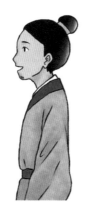
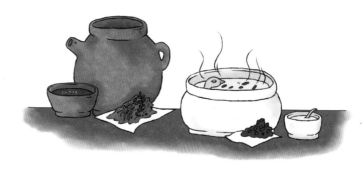

伊尹从汤羹中得到启发，在汤羹的基础上，发明了中药汤剂，使中药从生药变成熟药，并使用陶器煎煮草药为人治病，至此中药药效得到了大幅度提高。相传，伊尹还曾撰写《汤液经法》，奠定了中药方剂学的基础。

Inspired by the soup cooking, Yi Yin invented the traditional Chinese medicine decoction on the basis of the soup, which changed the traditional Chinese medicine from crude drug to processed medicine, and the pottery-cooked decoction greatly improved the efficacy of traditional Chinese medicine. According to record, Yi Yin also wrote *Decoction Method*, thus laying the foundation for the traditional Chinese medicine prescriptions.

虽然如今做汤的方式相较过往已大不相同，但伊尹制汤之法却在中药汤剂的煎煮中得以保留和延续，并在介于汤和汤剂之间的老火靓汤中得以再现。

The way of making soup today is quite different from that in the past, but Yi Yin's method has been preserved and developed in the process of decoction making. Moreover, it is re-adopted in cooking "Canton soup", the old fire soup between common soup and decoction.

# 煎药方式
## Decoction Making Approach

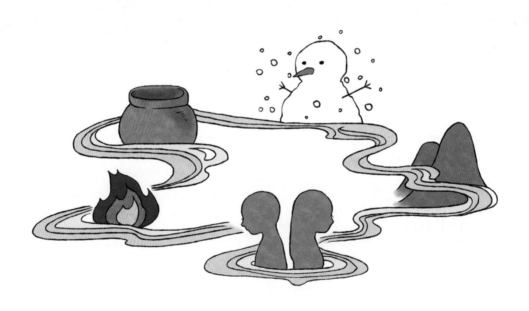

# 特点分析

老火靓汤制作的过程通常被称为煲汤，其制作也可看作是一种特殊的中药煎煮形式。与中药煎煮一样，老火靓汤的煲制对火候、炊具也有特殊要求。煲制时一般讲究先武火后文火，滋补靓汤煲制时间可长，而降火的靓汤时间则应短。同时煲汤时所用的炊具也应以砂锅为宜，从而使食材的滋味得以最大限度地渗入汤内。不仅如此，老火靓汤的选用同样须注重三因制宜，即因人、因时、因地制宜。如在炎热潮湿环境下，可选用薏米老鸭汤等清补降火的靓汤；而在寒冷的冬季或素体怕冷的人群，则可食用如当归生姜羊肉汤等温补的靓汤。

# Characteristic Analysis

The process of making soup is usually called boiling soup, and its cooking method can also be regarded as a special decoction form of traditional Chinese medicine. Like traditional Chinese medicine decoction, the cooking of soup has special requirement on heat and cooking utensils. For instance, it is better to use strong fire first, and then soft one. The cooking time of nourishing soup can be long, while the cooking time of soup for reducing fire should be short. Meanwhile, the cooking utensils should be casseroles, so that the taste of the ingredients can penetrate into the soup to the greatest extent. Plus, the choice of ingredients must also be relevant to three factors: people, season and region. In case in certain hot and humid area, some hot soup such as duck soup with coix seed would be a wise choice to decrease internal heat. But in the cold winter or for the people who are always afraid of the cold, hot soup such as mutton soup with angelica and ginger would be more appropriate for warming.

# 百药之长亦佳酿
## The Invention of Wine

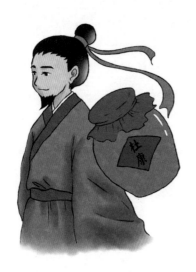

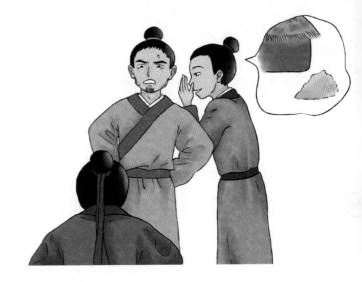

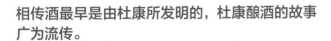

**相传酒最早是由杜康所发明的，杜康酿酒的故事广为流传。**

In China, wine is believed to have been invented by Du Kang, and his wine-brewing story is known to every household.

**上古时期大禹治理天下时，杜康负责看管粮仓。任职期间，杜康遭小人黄浪诬陷，因看管粮食霉变被逐还乡里。**

When Yu was the ruler of the country, Du Kang was in charge of the granary. During his term of office, Du Kang was framed by a villain Huang Lang for the moldy grains he was guarding, so he was deported back to his hometown.

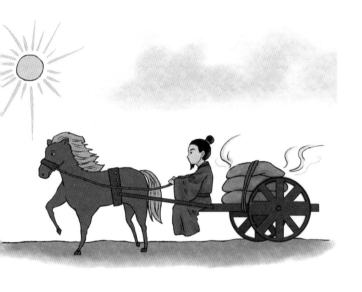

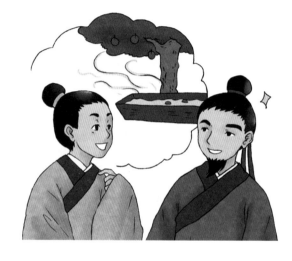

临行前，杜康到了粮库，闻见库外的霉粮中飘来一股奇异的香味，于是他特意装了几大包霉粮回家。

Before leaving, Du Kang went to the granary. There he smelt a strange fragrance coming from the moldy grains outside. Curiously, he packed several large bags of mildewy grains home.

一日，邻居来访，闻到霉粮的香味，竟说："这与我前日在果树下水槽中所闻到的香味十分相似，并且相当美味。"

One day, one of his neighbors came. He smelt the fragrance of moldy grains and said, "This one is very similar to the fragrance I smelt in the sink under the fruit tree the day before yesterday. It was quite delicious."

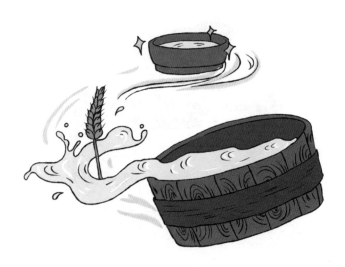

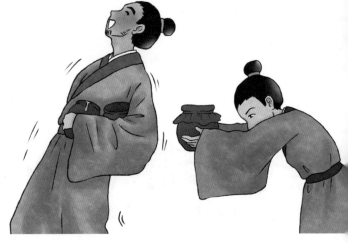

杜康听罢，心想这霉粮放入清水，说不定也能酿造出这样的水。经过不断尝试，杜康终于酿造出一种奇特之水，并在民间逐渐传了开来。

Du Kang took all his words in the heart. "Will the moldy grains be able to produce such liquid if kept in clean water?" He was wondering. After constant experiments, Du Kang finally brewed a peculiar liquid, which gradually gained popularity among the people.

黄浪听说此事后很是嫉妒，企图贪功，便将这奇特之水向大禹敬献。大禹饮后连声夸赞，但连饮数杯后却面目红赤，走路不稳，癫狂乱语。

Jealous for Du Kang's success, Huang Lang tried to take credit for the invention. He presented the liquid to Yu. After drinking, Yu repeatedly praised its taste. However, after several cups, he got red-faced, walking unsteadily and raving wildly.

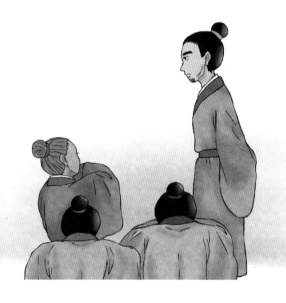

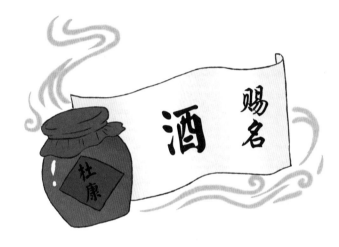

黄浪恐惧焦虑，企图再次嫁祸杜康。众大臣立即跪奏，成功为杜康雪冤。原来这奇特的水性烈，少喝可精神倍增，多喝却会眩晕失态。

Huang Lang, so terrified, again attempted to frame Du Kang. The ministers immediately knelt down to submit a written statement, successfully cleared him of the false charge. It turned out that this peculiar liquid was strong, and that drinking a small amount of it could cheer up the spirit, but a large amount could make you dizzy and even unconscious.

大禹赐这奇特之水以"酒"名，这便是"杜康酿酒"的传说，而杜康也成了酒的代名词。

Yu called this strange liquid "wine". And "Du Kang", the inventor's name, became a synonym for wine.

# 酒功效
## The Efficacy of Wine

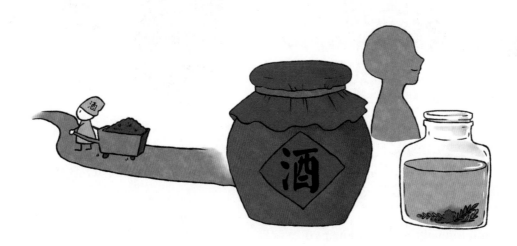

# 功效分析

酒是宴请餐桌上的常客，自古有"无酒不成宴"之说。在中医药领域，酒也有着广泛的应用，被誉为"百药之长"，繁体的"醫"字，其下半部"酉"字，便取自于酒。酒性温热，能够起到畅通血脉，散寒化瘀的作用。同时其又善行散，能行运药势，常可作为药媒促进其他药物到达病所，发挥治疗作用。因而，医圣张仲景以白酒作为药媒，配伍宣通胸阳的瓜蒌、薤白共同治疗胸痹（类似于冠心病、心绞痛）。在日常生活中，人们也常将一些具有保健功效的中药浸入酒中，每日小酌一杯，起到一定的养生保健作用。不过水能载舟亦能覆舟，无度饮酒不但会使人丧失理智，更会损害人的健康。

# Efficacy Analysis

Wine is frequently served in banquets. There goes a proverb "no wine, no feast". In the field of traditional Chinese medicine, wine, known as "the head of the medicines", is also widely used for medical treatment. The lower part of the traditional Chinese character "醫" (medicine) is "酉" (wine), which perfectly proves the relationship between wine and medicine. Wine is warm in nature. It can unblock blood vessels, dispel cold and remove blood stasis. At the same time, it is capable of transporting drugs. Hence, it is often used as a drug carrier to promote other drugs to reach disease sites and play a therapeutic role. Therefore, "Medical Sage" Zhang Zhongjing used wine as the drug carrier to treat thoracic obstruction (similar to coronary heart disease and angina pectoris) together with snakegourd fruit and *Allium macrostemon* which promote the release of yang in thorax. In daily life, people often dip some traditional Chinese medicine in the wine, hoping to gain some health care effect through it. However, as the water that bears the boat is the same that swallows it up, excessive drinking will not only make people lose their senses, but also harm health.

# 无意之举创豆腐
## Gypsum and Tofu

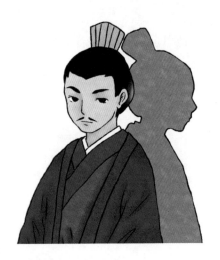

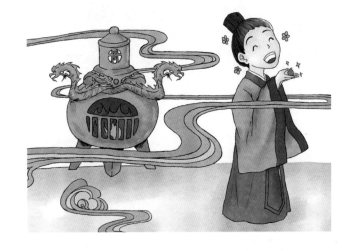

说到刘邦，恐怕无人不知无人不晓。但如果说刘邦之孙就知者甚少了，而他其实为中华饮食做出过一项杰出的贡献——那便是豆腐的发明。

Liu Bang, the first emperor of the Western Han Dynasty, is a household name. However, as for his grandson, few people have heard of his name. In fact, the grandson made an outstanding contribution to Chinese diet—the invention of tofu.

从秦汉至魏晋时期，炼丹追求长生不老之风盛行。而刘邦之孙淮南王刘安便是养生大军的一员。

From the Qin and Han Dynasties to the Wei and Jin, alchemy was popular in pursuit of immortality. The monarch of Huainan, Liu An, the grandson of Liu Bang, was a member of the health preservation chasers.

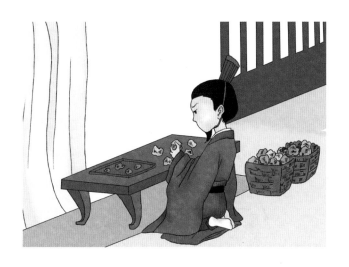

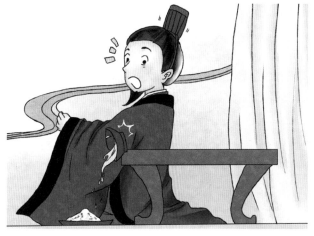

当时人们认为，自然界的矿石吸纳了天地精华，服石养生能够长生而不老，因而许多矿石类物质都被用来炼制长生不老的仙丹，这之中就包括石膏。

At that time, it was believed that natural minerals absorbed the essence of nature and that life expectancy could be extended by taking natural minerals, so many minerals were used to make immortal elixirs, including gypsum.

无巧不成书，刘安在一次炼丹过程中，无意间将热豆浆洒进了石膏之中。

During an alchemy, Liu An accidentally poured some hot soy-bean milk into the gypsum.

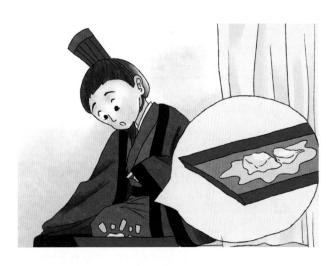

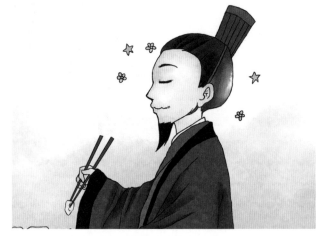

待他再去看时，神奇的事发生了，豆浆竟结成了块状。

When he returned, a miracle happened that the soybean milk became lumpy curd.

刘安认为这或许就是仙丹，便尝了一口，感觉十分美味。于是刘安虽炼丹求仙不成，却无心插柳促成了豆腐的诞生，而刘安也被誉为"豆腐的始祖"。

Thinking that might be the elixir, Liu An had a taste of it, "Whoa, so delicious!" Although Liu An failed his alchemy to immortality, he inadvertently contributed to the birth of tofu, earning himself "the father of tofu".

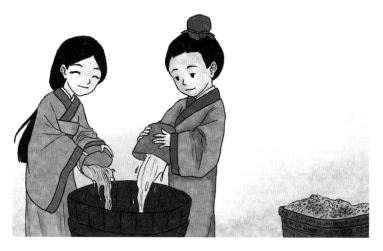

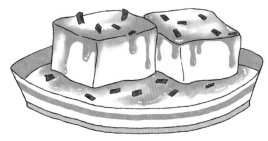

豆腐的制作工艺逐渐在民间流传开来，并得到完善发展。

至此，豆腐成了家家户户餐桌上不可或缺的美食，北京的小葱拌豆腐，扬州的文思豆腐便是其中的代表。

The technology for tofu production gradually spread widely among the people and was well developed afterwards.

Since then, tofu has become a daily food on every household's dining table, and two of the typical dishes with tofu are Peking tofu mixed with green onions and sliced tofu with mushrooms, ham and chicken by Monk Wensi in Yangzhou City.

# 石膏功效
## The Efficacy of Gypsum

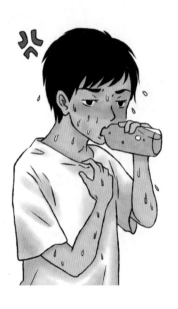

# 功效分析

在制作豆腐过程中，所用的石膏是煅石膏，而石膏在制作豆腐的过程中起收敛凝固的作用。其作为中药材，在治疗中所起的作用也是通过收敛的特性实现的。煅石膏的主要功效便是收湿敛疮，临床主要以外用为主，用于疮疡溃烂不敛、水火烫伤等病症。临床使用更为广泛的是生石膏。生石膏的最大特性在于其性大寒，清热力量强大，同时又兼具甘味，大寒可清热泻火，甘寒又可生津止渴，最适于临床高热不退、大汗淋漓、口干烦躁的患者。如医圣张仲景《伤寒论》中治疗高热不退的白虎汤便以生石膏为君药。

# Efficacy Analysis

In the process of making tofu, calcined gypsum is used for convergence and solidification. As a traditional Chinese medicine, gypsum also plays a role in treatment through convergence. The main effect of calcined gypsum is to astringe dampness and heal the wound. It is mainly used for external use in clinic for treating sore, ulcer, scald, etc. Hydrated gypsum is more widely used in clinic. Its best-known characteristic is its cold nature and strong heat-clearing power. Its cold nature can clear heat and purge fire, while its sweet taste and cold nature can promote fluid production and quench thirst, most suitable for patients with clinical high fever, profuse sweating, dry mouth and dysphoria. For example, according to *Treatise on Febrile Diseases* written by the Medical Sage Zhang Zhongjing, hydrated gypsum is the monarch drug for Bai Hu decoction, which is expected to treat high fever.

# 第二部分
# 寓药之情

中药在传统文化中并非只是治病的工具，同时它也被古人寄予了丰富的情感。

# Part II
# The Feelings in the Medicine

Traditional Chinese medicine is not only a mixture of substances for curing diseases in traditional culture, but also an embodiment of rich feelings and great love in ancient times.

# 母慈子孝益母草

## Motherwort and Filial Piety

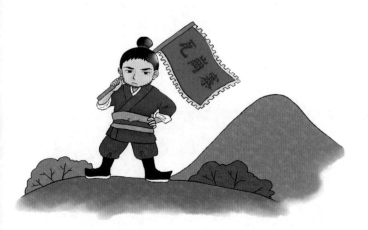

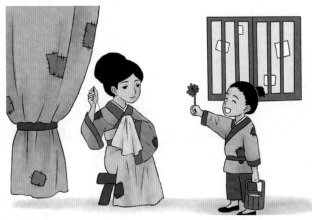

程咬金是隋唐时期赫赫有名的瓦岗寨首领，同时他也是一位不折不扣的孝子，中药益母草的命名便是源自于他。

Cheng Yaojin was a famous leader of Wagang Village in Sui and Tang Dynasties; meanwhile he was also a filial son. Motherwort, a kind of the traditional Chinese medicine, the name of which is related to him.

相传，程咬金幼年丧父，与母亲相依为命，家中一贫如洗。

According to legend, Cheng Yaojin was born in a poor family. His father died when he was very young. He lived a difficult life with his mother.

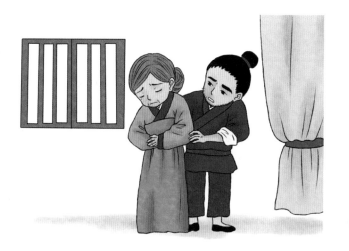

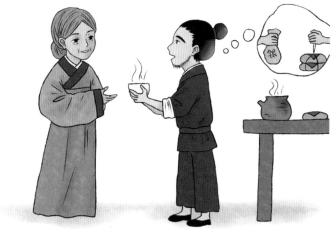

程母在生程咬金时，留下了产后瘀血疼痛的病。程咬金长大成人后，决心医好母亲的病。

When Cheng's mother gave birth to Cheng Yaojin, she suffered from postpartum blood stasis and felt painful all the time. When Cheng Yaojin grew up, he was determined to cure her disease.

程咬金拿着平日节省的碎银，到邻村郎中处给母亲配了两剂中药。吃了草药后，病情果然有所好转。

From the neighboring village doctor, Cheng Yaojin bought two doses of medicine with the hard-earned pennies he had saved. After taking the herbal medicine, his mother felt better.

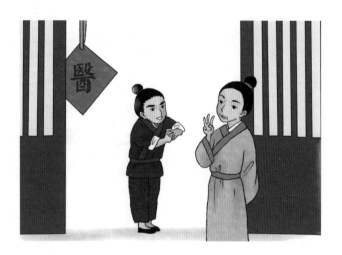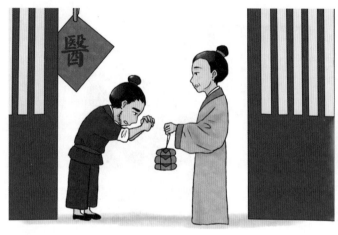

程咬金高兴极了，又跑去找那位郎中，而郎中说
这次得花三两银子。

Cheng Yaojin was so happy that he ran all the way to
the doctor asking for more medicine. However, the
doctor this time began to raise the price. "Three taels
of silver," he asked.

程咬金面露难色。忽然他灵机一动，答应等母亲
病愈后还钱。郎中同意了他的要求。

Cheng Yaojin looked slightly pained. Suddenly he got
an idea that he promised to pay back the money after
his mother's full recovery. The doctor agreed.

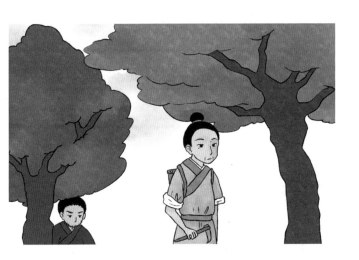

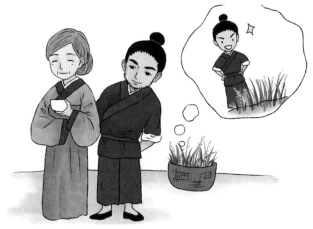

一日，郎中上山采药，程咬金便躲在后头偷偷跟着，看郎中采的是什么药，长在什么地方。

One day, the doctor went to collect herbs in the mountain. Cheng Yaojin followed him without being noticed. He remembered the herbs the doctor collected and the place where the herbs grew.

心里有数后，程咬金便自己到山里采来那种药，煎汤给母亲治病，终于把母亲病治好了。这药因此得名"益母草"。

Then Cheng Yaojin made the medicine by himself and finally cured his mother. Therefore, this medicine got the name "motherwort" from Cheng's story.

# 益母草功效
## The Efficacy of Motherwort

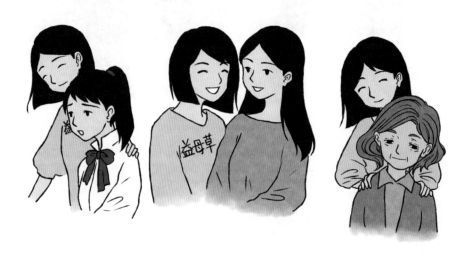

# 功效分析

益母草在多种妇科疾病中均有广泛的应用，如故事中程咬金母亲所患的产后瘀血疾病，益母草能活血化瘀，可有效应用于产后恶露未尽引起的腹痛；对于瘀血引起的月经不调，益母草能活血通经，调经止痛；同时，对于瘀血热毒引起的斑疹，益母草亦能活血化瘀，清热解毒，起到美容养颜的作用。"益母"之名可谓实至名归。

# Efficacy Analysis

The motherwort is widely used in various gynecological diseases. As in the case of postpartum blood stasis suffered by Cheng Yaojin's mother, motherwort could promote blood circulation and remove blood stasis and was effectively applied to abdominal pain caused by incomplete postpartum lochia. At the same time, for irregular menstruation caused by blood stasis, motherwort can promote blood circulation and dredge channels, regulate menstruation and relieve pain. Besides, motherwort can also clear away heat and toxic materials, and play the role of beauty for macula caused by blood stasis and toxic heat. The medicine "Yi Mu ('Yi' means 'good for' and 'Mu' means 'mother' or 'female' in Chinese)" indeed deserves its name.

# 待客之道槟榔礼
## *Areca catechu* and Courtesy

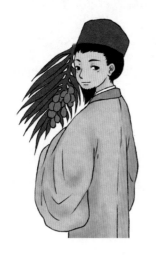

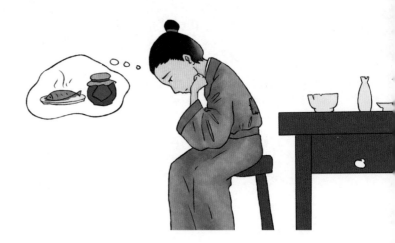

刘穆之是南朝宋的一位大臣。在开国皇帝刘裕北伐期间，他曾屡次留守都城，掌管朝廷内外事务，被誉为"刘宋"的第一号功臣。不过，他年轻时却异常落魄。

Liu Muzhi was a minister of the Song of the Southern Dynasty. During the Northern Expedition led by the Founding Emperor Liu Yu, he stayed in the capital city several times and managed both internal and external affairs for the imperial court. Due to his talent and achievement, he was praised as the No.1 hero of "Liu Song Period". Though greatly honored, Liu Muzhi was extremely down and out when he was young.

年轻时的他十分贫穷，经常是衣不蔽体，食不果腹。但他却特别喜爱酒食。

Liu used to live in great poverty, unable to wear warm or feed himself. Ironically, he very much lusted after wine and food!

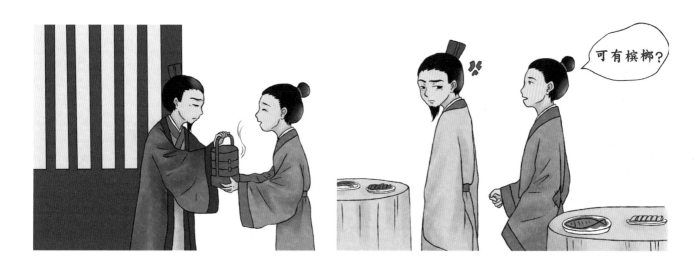

娶妻之后，因为他的妻兄家境相对富裕，于是他便时常去妻兄家里蹭吃蹭喝。妻兄也是无可奈何。

After marriage, he often went to his brother-in-law's house for free food and wine, for the latter was relatively rich. The brother-in-law could do nothing but accept him.

有一次，妻兄家里办喜事，刘穆之又是不请自来。饭后，刘穆之仍不满足，又向妻兄要槟榔来消食。

One day, his brother-in-law was holding a wedding. As usual, Liu Muzhi came uninvited. After dinner, still unsatisfied, Liu Muzhi asked his brother-in-law for *Areca catechu* to help digestion.

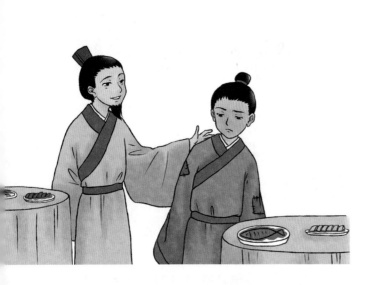

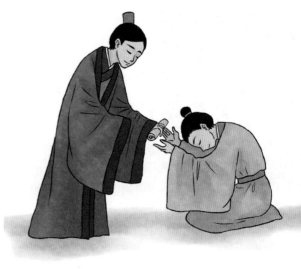

妻兄便讽刺他说："既然你经常挨饿，又需要这消食的槟榔来做什么呢？"

"Since you often go hungry, why do you need this *Areca catechu* for digestion?" his brother-in-law satirized him.

时来运转，刘穆之后来得到了刘裕的赏识，跟随刘裕南征北战，并担任了丹阳尹。

Later Liu Muzhi won the appreciation of Emperor Liu Yu, following him everywhere and serving as the magistrate of Danyang City.

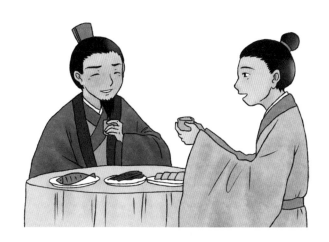

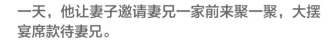

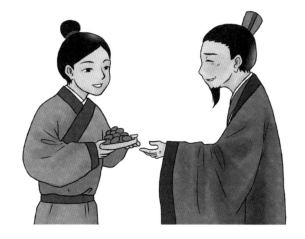

一天，他让妻子邀请妻兄一家前来聚一聚，大摆宴席款待妻兄。

One day, he asked his wife to invite her brother's family to banquet.

酒足饭饱之后，刘穆之便让人用金盘装满槟榔拿给妻兄。妻兄想到之前对刘穆之的讥讽，顿时感到羞愧万分。

At the end of the banquet, Liu Muzhi had the *Areca catechu* served on gold plates and presented it to his brother-in-law. Immediately after he recalled the previous sarcasm to Liu Muzhi, did he feel extremely ashamed.

# 槟榔功效
## The Efficacy of *Areca catechu*

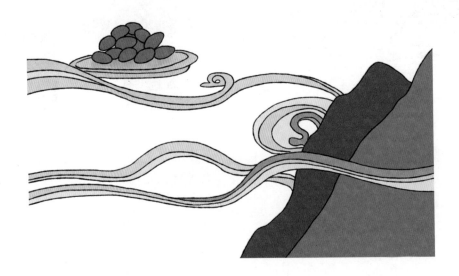

# 功效分析

我国岭南地区气候炎热潮湿，常阻遏脾胃运化，并易导致食物腐败，引起如食欲不振、肠道寄生虫疾病等消化道病症。刘穆之饭后嚼槟榔的习惯便与槟榔的消食作用有关。同时槟榔又可杀虫驱虫，用于多种肠道寄生虫疾病。另外，对于湿浊引起的脚气肿痛，槟榔尚能行气利水。因而在岭南地区，槟榔不仅是可口的零食，还是一味能够防病治病的良药。不仅如此，岭南人更是有"客至不设茶，唯以槟榔为礼"的传统，将槟榔作为待客的礼节、礼品。可见槟榔早已成为了当地文化的一部分。

# Efficacy Analysis

The hot and humid climate in Lingnan region of our country often inhibits the digestion and absorption of spleen and stomach, and easily leads to food corruption, causing digestive tract diseases such as anorexia and intestinal parasitic diseases. Liu Muzhi's habit of chewing *Areca catechu* after meals was precisely related to its efficacy in helping digestion. In addition, *Areca catechu* can also kill and repel insects, and can be used for various intestinal parasitic diseases. Besides, *Areca catechu* can promote flow of qi and urination for swelling and pain of beriberi caused by turbid dampness. Being a good medicine, *Areca catechu* is also a delicious snack. Lingnan people even have the custom of treating guests with *Areca catechu* instead of tea, making *Areca catechu* a courtesy gift. *Areca catechu* has become part of local culture.

# 闭门逐客王不留

## *Vaccaria segetalis* and Deportation Order

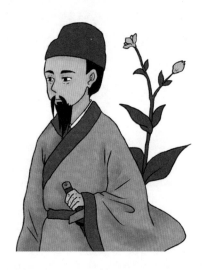

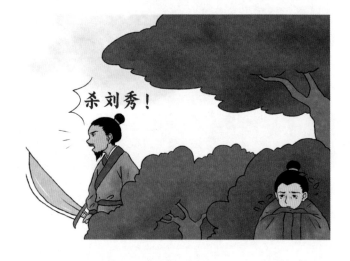

邳彤为东汉开国功臣，名列云台二十八将之一。同时，他还钟情于中草药材，精通医药。相传王不留行便是由他命名的。

Pi Tong was one of the 28 generals in Yuntai who made great contributions to the founding of the Eastern Han Dynasty. Besides those achievements in his official career, he also loved Chinese herbal medicine and was proficient in it. It is said that "Wangbuliuxing" (*Vaccaria segetalis*) was named by him.

西汉末年，王莽自封为王，率兵追杀刘秀，认为他才是汉室后裔，企图以新朝取代西汉。

In the later Western Han Dynasty, Wang Mang proclaimed himself the emperor and led his troops to kill Liu Xiu. He believed that he himself was the legal descendant of the Han Dynasty, so he attempted to replace the Western Han Dynasty with a new one.

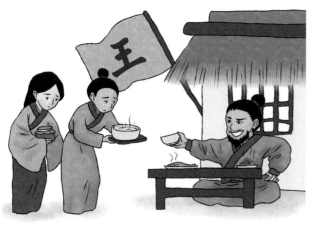

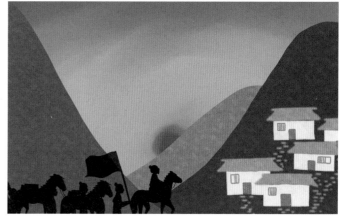

王莽的部队每到一个地方便抢占老百姓的房子，还要求老百姓给他们送饭菜，百姓怨声载道。

Wherever Wang Mang's troops went, they occupied the houses of the common people and commanded them to offer food to them. So people everywhere complained.

一日黄昏，王莽的部队来到邳彤的故乡。眼见天黑，王莽却见全村家家关门锁户，没有一缕炊烟。

One day, Wang Mang's troops reached the hometown of Pi Tong at dusk. To his great surprise, he saw all the doors in the village were closed and that no one was cooking.

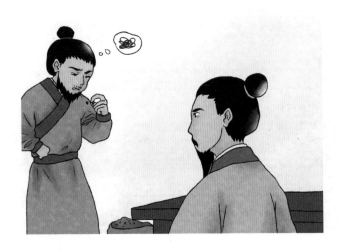

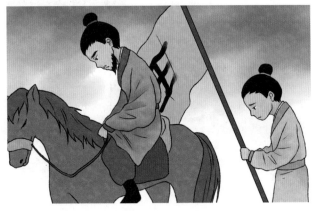

此时只有邳彤守在家中，但家中没有米粮，只有一种植物的种子。王莽拿了一粒放在嘴里，口味苦涩，便慌忙吐了出来。

Pi Tong was the only one staying at home. However, there was no rice in his stove but a kind of seeds. Wang Mang took one and put it in his mouth. It tasted bitter, so he threw it up in a hurry.

眼见村中得不到便宜，王莽只能带着部队气鼓鼓、灰溜溜地离开了。

Seeing that he could get nothing from the village, Wang Mang left with his troops in disgrace.

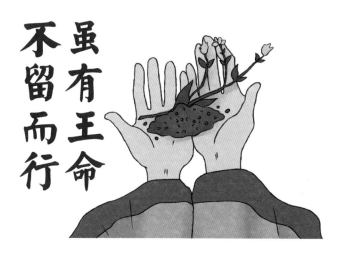

不留而行 虽有王命

事后，邳彤给这种子起名王不留行，以寓意"虽有王命，不留而行"之义，同时也告诫后人"得民心者，得天下"的道理。

Afterwards, Pi Tong named the seed "Wangbuliuxing", implying "In spite of the emperor's order (Wang), you might as well leave (Buliuxing)". Meanwhile, Pi Tong warned the later generations of the truth that "those who have the people's heart, have the world".

# 王不留行功效
## The Efficacy of *Vaccaria segetalis*

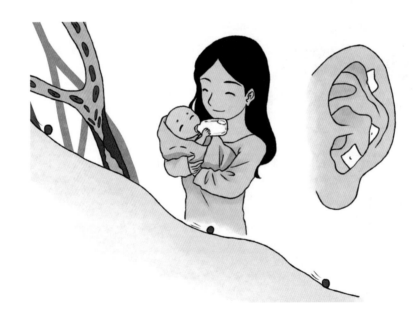

# 功效分析

王不留行字面上的意思便带有逐客的意味，而作为药用亦是药如其名，其药性可以一个"通"字来概括。在中医理论中，关于疼痛有着"不通则痛"的观点。当经脉不通畅，瘀血形成，便会导致疼痛的发生，王不留行能够通经活血以缓解瘀滞引起的疼痛。同时，在民间流传着"穿山甲、王不留，妇人食了乳长流"的顺口溜。对于哺乳期妇女乳汁积滞或者乳汁不畅引起的奶结、少乳，王不留行具有通经下乳的作用。另外，王不留行的通达之性还被用于耳穴的治疗中，能够刺激穴位，增强疗效。

# Efficacy Analysis

Wangbuliuxing can be thought as "a deportation order" literally. As a medicine, Wangbuliuxing has such efficacy as well. Its property can be summarized into one word "unblockage". In the theory of traditional Chinese medicine, there is a point of view that pain is caused by obstruction. When the meridians are not smooth and blood stasis is formed, it will lead to the occurrence of pain. Wangbuliuxing can pass the meridians and activate blood to relieve the pain caused by stagnation. At the same time, there is a popular saying among the civilians that "Pangolin, *Vaccaria segetalis*, women can vigorously secrete milk after taking". For lactating women with milk stagnation or poor milk caused by the milk knot, less milk, Wangbuliuxing has the role of dredging and promoting milk secretion. In addition, Wangbuliuxing's property of "unblockage" is also used in the treatment of auricular points by stimulating the acupoints, thus enhancing the curative effect.

# 志存高远誉远志
## Polygala and Aspiration

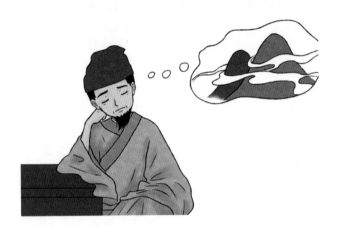

东晋时期，谢安高卧东山，隐居山林至四十余岁，不愿出仕。

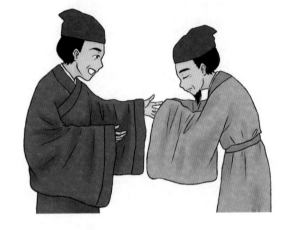

后来官府征召的命令多次下达，让他出山为官，势不得已，谢安才答应出山，就任桓温属下的司马。

During the Eastern Jin Dynasty, lived in the Dongshan Mountains an over 40-year-old scholar Xie An, who was reclusive and unwilling to serve in the imperial court.

Later, after having been repeatedly sent government conscription orders requesting him to serve as an official, Xie An reluctantly went out of the mountains and became minister under the command of Huan Wen.

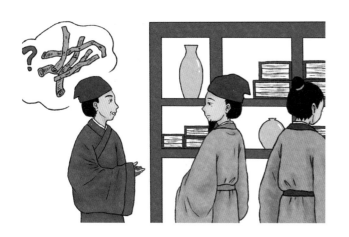

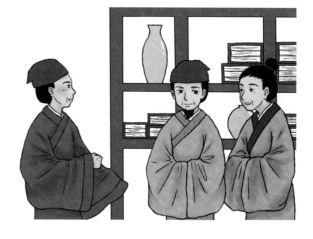

谢安去拜见桓温时，有人送草药给桓温，其中有远志。桓温见物起意，便拿来问谢安："这种药又被称为小草，为什么同一种药却有两种名称呢？"

When Xie An went to visit Huan Wen, Huan Wen showed him some polygala he had been given before. He asked Xie An,"As far as I know, this medicine is also called grass. Why does the same medicine have two different names?"

谢安没有立即回答。当时郝隆在座，随声回答说："这很容易解释啊，不出（隐居）就是远志，出（出仕）就是小草。"谢安听后，知道郝隆是在讥讽自己素有远志，出山却只做一个小小的司马，不由脸上露出了惭愧之色。

Xie An was just about to answer when Hao Long, who was present, replied, "The reason is simple. If you stay in the mountains (in seclusion), you are polygala; and if you go to the court (in official positions), you are grass." Immediately Xie An understood Hao Long was mocking himself for the embarrassing situation that despite of his great ambition, he now ended with a low-ranked minister. Xie An could do nothing but feel shameful for himself.

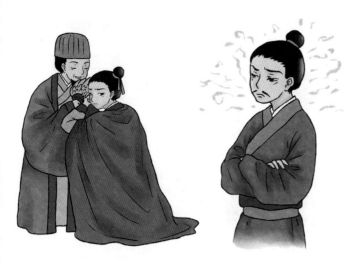

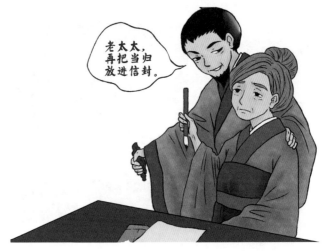

建兴六年，魏国天水郡太守马遵对姜维极不友善，怀疑他对魏国有异心，姜维便毅然投靠诸葛亮。

In the sixth year of Jianxing, Ma Zun, Governor of Tianshui County of Wei State, was extremely unfriendly to Jiang Wei. Being suspected of his disloyalty to Wei State, Jiang Wei finally decided to turn to Zhuge Liang.

魏国的谋臣知道姜维是一个不可多得的人才，便又想方设法争取他"回归"。他们知道姜维是个孝子，便将他母亲接到洛阳，诱逼她写信给姜维，并在信封里附上当归，其意要姜维回归魏国。

One of Wei's advisers knew Jiang Wei was a rare talent, so he tried every means to win his "return". Knowing that Jiang Wei was a filial son, he had his mother brought to Luoyang, inducing her to write to Jiang Wei. Also he enclosed the envelope with angelica, the Chinese name of which meant "return back".

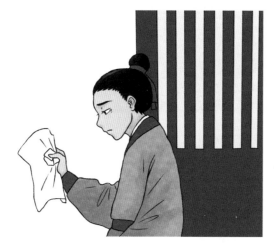

但有远志
不在当归

姜维收到信后，明白其意。他反复思量后做出了自己的抉择——决定继续效忠蜀国。于是他给母亲回信，并附上了远志。他含泪写道："良田百顷，不在一亩（母）；但有远志，不在当归。"

When receiving the letter, Jiang Wei fully understood the implied meaning. After a second thought, he made his own decision to continue his loyalty to Shu State. So he wrote back to his mother, and attached it with polygala. Tearfully he said in his letter, "There are a hundred hectares of fertile land here, so I do not care about an acre (homophonic to 'mother' in Chinese); There is polygala（'great ambition' in Chinese）in my heart, so I will not return back."

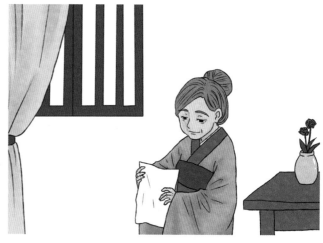

知子莫若母，姜母接到儿子的信，理解地说道："儿有远志，母无它求。"于是姜母便一头撞死，以绝姜维的牵挂。

After reading the letter, Jiang's mother said understandably, "As a son has high aspiration, can a mother expect any more of him?" In order to cut off her son's worries, Jiang's mother committed suicide by hitting her head on the wall.

# 远志功效
## The Efficacy of Polygala

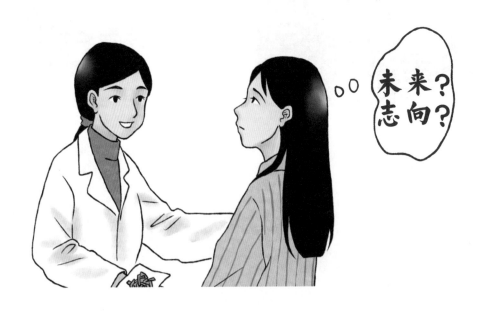

# 功效分析

郝隆以远志小草讽刺谢安缺乏志向，而姜维则以远志来表明自己的心迹。远志，其名称独特的文学内涵也成了历代有识之士明志上进的象征。作为药用，远志也是药如其名，确有其效，能够益智安神、益智强记，具有使人聪颖、治疗健忘的功效。

# Efficacy Analysis

Hao Long used "Grass" instead of "Yuan Zhi" (polygala) to satirize Xie An's lack of ambition, while Jiang Wei showed his heart with polygala. Polygala, whose name is unique in its literary connotation, has also become a symbol of the aspiration of intelligent people. As its name tells, polygala can improve intelligence, soothe the nerves, treat amnesia by helping patients with their memory and intelligence.

食可療疾名傳修
品味本草怪藥心
飲湯斟酒岂佳餚
寓藥於食享康尋
盡孝言誌待客祺
康下藥君有情香